HEALING YOUR THYROID DISORDER NATURALLY!

End the frustration and learn what your doctor doesn't know.

Dr. Michael C. Taggart D.C.

HEALING YOUR THYROID DISORDER NATURALLY!

Dr. Michael C. Taggart D.C.

Michael C. Taggart, DC

11656 98th Ave. NE Suite B

Kirkland, WA 98034

425-821-1101

www.kirklandhealthinstitute.com

Limits of Liability and Disclaimer of Warranty:

Do you want to learn more about Dr. Taggart's practice and healing techniques? Please go to http://kirklandhealthinstitute.com/

If you are interested in visiting Dr. Taggart's office for an initial consultation, please call 425-821-1101. If you live in an area beyond Seattle, WA, USA, a phone or Skype consultation can be scheduled.

"I'm finally getting results! I've been struggling for a long time with thyroid issues, adrenal fatigue, anemia, Hashimoto's, inflammation, and chronic neck pain. After many disappointing visits with multiple doctors, including holistic practitioners, I found Dr. Taggart. Dr. Taggart quickly diagnosed my symptoms and created a simple program that I can follow with minimal effort that is producing outstanding results.

"I'm experiencing more energy, less pain, increased brain function, better balance, and I'm finally losing weight! And the neck and back adjustments are astounding! I'm so glad to have found Dr. Taggart. It feels so good to finally know exactly what to do to regain my health. Stop suffering and go see Dr. Taggart."

Katherine S., Snoqualmie, WA

Dedication

I'm dedicating this book to all the patients who over the years it has been a privilege to serve. Thank you for your faith in me. Thank you for believing that by working together we can conquer any problem! You have taught me so much, and have inspired me to be a better doctor.

Two special acknowledgements:

To Michael L. Johnson DC, DACBN for introducing me to functional neurology and continually motivating me and all the member doctors of the neuro-metabolic-super group to be the best and to never stop believing in ourselves.

To my wife Juli, for all your love and support.

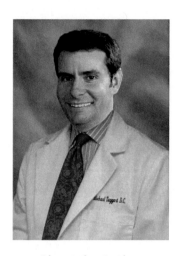

About the Author

Dr. Michael Taggart practices in Kirkland Washington USA. He has been in practice for over twenty years and specializes in helping patients overcome chronic health conditions. Dr. Taggart combines comprehensive neurological and metabolic testing to find the underlying causes of chronic conditions. Advanced neurologic therapies and specific nutritional protocols are used to allow the body to more fully heal itself. Dr. Taggart is an expert in functional medicine, having taken numerous postgraduate courses in functional neurology, functional endocrinology, and nutritional therapy.

Preface

Twenty-seven million Americans, and millions more worldwide, suffer with thyroid illness. Unfortunately, thyroid dysfunction is often missed by many doctors even when patients' complaints are classically thyroid; this happens due to lack of knowledge, inadequate testing, and using out-of-date lab ranges. Dr. Michael Taggart has done a masterful job in explaining what patients need to do to understand their symptoms, get the right tests done, and find an expert who has the training to turn their condition around. If you have thyroid symptoms, you need to read this book! You will find his book understandable and immensely valuable on your journey for better health.

Michael C. Johnson, DC, DACNB

Author of *You Can Beat Thyroid Disorders!* and *What Do You Do When the Medications Don't Work, A Non-Drug Treatment of Dizziness, Migraine Headaches, Fibromyalgia, and Other Chronic Conditions.*

Table of Contents

Chapter 1. Why Do I Feel So Bad?

And why can't anyone find out what's wrong with me?

These are all-too-familiar questions that I hear from patients, when they have been to multiple doctors with little to no improvement. The symptoms, mostly women report are these:

Fatigue

General feeling of cold all over/cold hands and feet

Hair that is thinning/falling out

Constipation/irritable bowel symptoms

Can't lose any weight, even on a low-calorie diet

Depression/anxiety

Outer one-third of the eyebrow thinning

Dry skin

Require excessive amount of sleep to function properly

Mental sluggishness

Muscle achiness

Morning headaches that wear off as the day goes by

Do these symptoms sound familiar?

You may not have all these symptoms, but if you have three to four there is a good chance your thyroid gland may be involved.

Before we talk specifically about these symptoms and the thyroid, let's talk about the health of the American population in general.

If you're following any media sources, newspaper, blogs, magazines, etc. you know it's not good. The World Health Organization studied the one hundred health care systems of all the industrialized nations and reported their findings. They rated the United States as one of the best systems for crisis care (i.e. you have a heart attack, stroke, massive injury, acute infection).

Our system is one of the best at saving your life in a crisis. Unfortunately our whole system is based on crisis intervention with drugs and surgery, but it does not effectively address the causes of why people develop disease in the first place.

According to the U.N. report, seventy-six countries that spend far less than the United States actually have healthier people! The study said the United States ranks forty-ninth in life expectancy, first in health care costs. We are paying more for living shorter lives! WHO researchers said, "Basically, you die earlier and spend more time disabled if you're an American rather than a member of most other advanced countries." [1]

> Two trillion dollars are spent on healthcare each year in the United States; we are only 3 percent of the world's population, yet we consume 60 percent of all manufactured drugs. You would think we would have some of the healthiest people in the world; unfortunately the exact opposite is true.

With ever-increasing costs and poor long-term health outcomes, we have created an insurance crisis in our country, creating a major economic burden on families, companies and government all trying to find solutions to keep people insured.

We live in a society where our food is overly processed, depleting the available nutrients our bodies need to function. In addition, there have been huge increases in sugar consumption in the American diet. Obesity is a national problem as well as the related rapid increase in the number of people developing diabetes. We have genetically modified foods, which are engineered to absorb more pesticides. Animal livestock are fed antibiotics and hormones to increase weight rapidly. When we consume their dairy and meat products, we absorb these drug residues (called xenobiotics and xenoestrogens). It's no wonder with all the dietary, economic, and social stresses that we have to deal with that the adaptive mechanisms of the body have been under assault! Have you heard of the S.A.D. diet? It's also known as "Standard American Diet;" now you know why: It's promoting poor health and disease.

As a result of the declining health of Americans, autoimmunity is one of the fastest growing conditions, affecting sixteen million Americans. One in twelve women now have autoimmunity, 1 in 25 men are affected. Autoimmunity may likely be the key to helping you understand your symptoms and why despite seeing many doctors you have not improved.

Chapter 2. What Does My Thyroid Do in My Body?

Every cell in your body depends on thyroid hormone function.

The small, bean-sized gland that lies behind your Adam's apple is very important indeed. You cannot live without thyroid hormones and cannot hope to have a good energy level without your thyroid working at an optimal level. The thyroid gland is like a pilot light for a furnace. When it gets cold in the house, the pilot light will ignite the furnace and the increased heat will warm the house. If your thyroid is low functioning there is not enough circulating hormone to bring oxygen and energy into the cells, keeping your body warm and energetic. Many people with thyroid problems, the majority of which are women, complain of low energy and feeling cold, among other symptoms. The thyroid is part of your endocrine system, each part of which works together to regulate all your hormones.

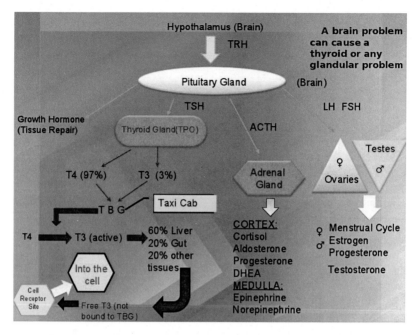

There is a lot going on in this chart, but don't get overwhelmed. We will take this step by step.

A gland in your brain called the hypothalamus monitors the level of thyroid hormone in the bloodstream. When thyroid hormones decrease, the hypothalamus will stimulate the pituitary gland with thyroid releasing hormone (TRH), and then the pituitary will stimulate the thyroid through thyroid stimulating hormone (TSH), which will cause the thyroid to make thyroid hormones. The body needs four and three molecules of iodine to produce T4 and T3. These are your thyroid hormones. As the level of thyroid hormones rises in a feedback loop mechanism the levels of TRH and TSH will decrease.

The pituitary is called the "master gland" because not only does it modulate thyroid hormone production but it also stimulates the other endocrine gland as well!

The pituitary also stimulates the adrenal glands through adrenal corticotropic hormone (ACTH). The adrenal gland has two parts: the cortex which produces cortisol, aldosterone, some progesterone and estrogen, and DHEA; and in the adrenal medulla, where epinephrine and norepinephrine are made. These substances help you adapt to stress. There is a similar feedback loop between the pituitary and the adrenal glands.

The pituitary also regulates the hormones of the reproductive system through a feedback system by producing follicle stimulating hormone (FSH) and luteinizing hormone (LH). FSH stimulates estrogen production, and LH produces progesterone in the female reproductive system.

In the male FSH stimulates spermatogenesis, and LH stimulates testosterone production.

Take away: All the endocrine glands interact with each other; a dysfunction in one gland leads to problems in others and even in the whole system. Clinically, the entire system needs to be evaluated to make sure that any intervention is appropriate. Failure to do this will lead to poor results and unintended side-effects.

Now once thyroid hormones are produced, it is important to follow how they get to the tissue cells and how gut and liver function influence this process. When thyroid hormones are produced, a large percentage become bound to thyroid-binding globulins, or TBGs. The TBG and other binding globulins are proteins that are made by the liver. Only a small percentage of the thyroid hormones remain free floating in the blood stream, and *only the free-floating hormones can hook onto cell receptor sites and produce a biological effect in the body.* Once a thyroid hormone is bound to the protein (TBGs), it is bound forever. The TBGs are like a taxicab that allows you to get in and drives you all over town but never allows you to exit the vehicle! The body uses the binding globulins as a way to safeguard against having too many thyroid hormones (or other hormones), which can create a hyperthyroid state (dangerous to the heart).

Another important point, is that the thyroid produces 94 percent T4 and only 3 percent T3. T4 is mostly biologically inactive so we have only free-floating T3 to get to the cells. That is not nearly enough thyroid hormone for the whole body! So the body has to convert some of the T4 into T3, and it does this by using the liver, gut and the peripheral tissues (muscles, bones etc.) to make more free T3.

If your liver and or gastrointestinal systems are compromised, you can develop a thyroid problem. (I will talk more about the gut and the liver in future chapters.)

Now that you know that poor thyroid function can affect just about every system of the body, let's make a more comprehensive list of what thyroid dysfunction can affect.

The thyroid, along with the parathyroid, controls calcium absorption and can lead to weak bones and osteoporosis.

The thyroid stimulates the bowels and when deficient can cause constipation and interfere with HCL production in the stomach, leading to malabsorption, bloating, heartburn, and leaky gut syndrome.

Thyroid hormone is important for liver and gall bladder function. A deficiency can lead to high cholesterol or triglycerides. Blood sugar imbalances are a factor here as well in raising cholesterol and triglycerides.

Low thyroid function interferes with fertility.

Anemia can be a result of low thyroid function.

Protein synthesis is affected by low thyroid hormone levels, producing reduced muscle mass, dry skin, hair loss, and impaired healing in general.

Low thyroid affects brain function and mood by inhibiting frontal lobe activity and impairing serotonin, dopamine, and GABA neurotransmitter metabolism.

Low thyroid slows your metabolism causing weight gain, and an inability to lose weight even on a low calorie-diet.

Take away: *In order for the thyroid hormones to enter the cells they have to be converted to the active form T3. Every cell in your body has a receptor site for thyroid hormones; this explains why so many symptoms can result from poor thyroid function.*

Chapter 3. The #1 Reason Why People Have a Chronic Thyroid Problem

It's probably not what you think.

According to the most up-to-date research, approximately 90 percent of patients with hypothyroidism have it as a result of an autoimmune reaction called Hashimoto's Thyroiditis.

Hashimoto's is the most common autoimmune condition affecting twenty-four million Americans, or 7 to 8 percent of the population. [2] [3]

Autoimmunity occurs when the immune system becomes imbalanced and attempts to destroy your body tissues by mistake. There is a subtle balance between not enough immune response and too much response.

Let's talk about basic immune function to help you understand the problem. In your body you have a part of the immune system that destroys cells; it's called the TH1 system or T cells. Let's call that part of the immune system the "SWAT team." Some of the names of the cells in this system are "cytotoxic killer cells;" you get the idea. The other side of the immune system is the TH2 system, or B cells, some of the names of these cells are T-helper cells and T-regulatory cells. This part of the immune system puts a target, or antibody when necessary on invading and abnormal cells so that the SWAT team (TH1) can find the bad guys and take them out. To have a healthy immune system the TH1 and TH2 sides of the immune system must be balanced. When one side becomes more dominant things start going wrong, causing an inappropriate response.

For example if the TH1 system becomes overactive the swat team is going to go overboard and take out tissues that it shouldn't be destroying. If the TH2 system becomes dominate then the immune system would be overdoing it by putting a tag (antibody) on tissues that it shouldn't be targeting for destruction by the TH1 cells. Either way we have unwanted cell destruction.

The third part of the immune system is the TH3 and TH17 system. This part of the immune system, if functioning properly, helps keep the TH1 and TH2 systems from tilting into dominance either way.

This diagram will help you see the big picture of the immune system.

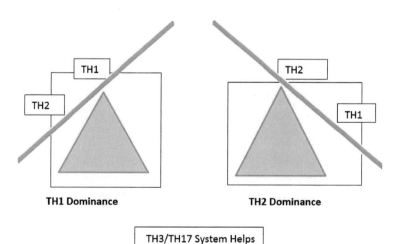

Chapter 4. What Causes Autoimmunity?

Why did I develop an Autoimmune Condition?

If you have an autoimmune condition, it's because you have a genetic predisposition to develop this disorder based on your inherited genes. This does not mean that those characteristics will always manifest. You have to experience the second part to develop autoimmunity, the triggers!

Important point: I always ask my patients on the first visit, "Does anyone else in your family that is a blood relative have similar problems? The mother, grandmother, aunt, or uncle, etc.?" If they have similar symptoms or another named autoimmune condition or were just chronically ill but no diagnosis was ever given, *this is a strong indication of how autoimmunity runs in families.*

For example, my stepfather has four daughters. His youngest daughter was diagnosed with celiac disease, which is an autoimmune disorder of the colon where the genes are not present to digest gluten. Because of this diagnosis, her two children were tested and diagnosed with celiac disease as well. My stepfather's oldest daughter, Caryn, started experiencing chronic fatigue and chronic pain in her fifties; with my guidance she was able to find the right doctors and discovered that she had celiac disease as well. Their grandmother suffered with chronic health problems but was never given any diagnoses, but it was suggested that she might have lupus which is another auto-immune disorder. Due to these findings, my stepfather's other two daughters have been checked and do not have celiac disease.

To develop autoimmunity you have to have the second piece of the equation: the triggers!

There are several metabolic syndromes and exposures that will activate the autoimmune genes!

These are the major players:

Chronic infections. When you have an exposure to a microbe, your immune system will initiate a response and typically your immune system wins the battle. However, there are instances in which your immune system cannot defeat the microorganism. This can happen as a result of other conditions you have developed that would mitigate a proper immune response. (We will discuss some of these issues below.)

Digestive problems. Eighty percent of your immune system is found in the gut. Low hydrochloric acid, constipation/diarrhea, and gas bloating are all signs that your gut is unhealthy. The chronic infections are often found here, which eventually will damage the lining of the intestines, causing a leaky gut syndrome.

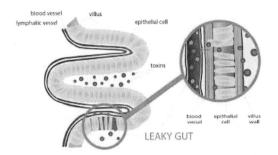

LEAKY GUT

Food allergies/sensitivity. The resulting inflammation of the leaky gut syndrome will cause undigested food proteins to slip past the barrier in the intestinal lining. These proteins will be detected by the immune system and will be treated as invaders. The immune system will initiate a strong response, increasing inflammation, and will "remember" the next time you eat the same or similar foods, aggravating the problem over and over again.

Low vitamin D. This vitamin is really a hormone and is one of the most important substances in the body. You can synthesize enough vitamin D without any dietary intake by direct sun exposure for twenty minutes. Unfortunately, with modern life we spend most of the day indoors and especially if you live in areas where there aren't a lot of sunny days, like where I live, in the Northwest, it can be a real problem. Every patient I see gets checked for vitamin D regardless of the complaint. Vitamin D is also an important part of the TH3 system, which helps keep TH1-TH2 dominance in check.

Blood sugar problems. Blood sugar problems are the #1 health problem affecting Americans. Diabetes and prediabetes (insulin resistance) are an epidemic in our country. When your diet is too rich in carbohydrates, especially grains, your body overproduces insulin. Over time the receptor sites for insulin that allow the blood sugar to get into the cell for energy stop responding to insulin, so the blood sugar stays in the blood stream, raising your levels. This will also increase your fat storage because the body will attempt to convert the blood sugar to fat and store it, increasing your waistline. Insulin is inflammatory, and inflammation damages the intestinal lining, impairs gland-to-gland communication, and further drives more immune imbalance.

Environmental toxins. Heavy metal and chemical exposure from pesticides, xenoestrogens, BPA from plastics, to name a few - these toxins are found abundantly in our society through the products we are exposed to, eat, or use.

Low levels of essential fatty acids. Every cell has a fatty layer around it. The brain is mostly made of fat; low fatty acid levels disrupt cell function and promote inflammation - Americans tend to be lacking omega 3 fatty acids. These oils are found in fish oil and some algaes and nuts, such as flax seeds, hemp seeds, chia seeds, walnuts, and for those limiting their fat intake, in leafy green vegetables.

Adrenal gland dysfunction. The adrenal gland sits on the top of the kidneys and performs many vital functions including sex hormone production (estrogen and testosterone through DHEA production) and progesterone in small quantities - The adrenal hormone aldosterone is involved in salt balance. Production of cortisol by the adrenal glands is involved in regulating the body's use of fats, proteins, and carbohydrates and is closely associated with blood sugar regulation. Cortisol has a big effect on sleep because it regulates melatonin, the sleep hormone made by the pineal gland. Your adrenal glands also make adrenaline (epinephrine) and noradrenaline (norepinephrine), which are substances that help you deal with stress. The factors that stress the adrenal glands are all the factors mentioned earlier.

Digestive inflammation

Chronic infections

Blood sugar imbalances

Food allergies

In addition, pain and emotional stress also affect the adrenal gland. Most of my patients have adrenal issues.

Chapter 5. Non-Autoimmune Thyroid Patterns

Six major metabolic pathways that can give you low thyroid symptoms without being autoimmune disorders.

As we have previously stated, the majority of thyroid problems have an autoimmune component to them. However, some thyroid problems are non-autoimmune. You may have only one or two of the autoimmune triggers, or you don't have a genetic susceptibility so you don't develop autoimmunity. We have talked about a number of the metabolic patterns in the last chapter. We will expand on them a little more and talk about what you would see on a blood test to determine which one of the seven patterns you have. You can have more than one pattern at a time. When you are autoimmune you will have several of these mechanisms occurring at the same time.

Before we go over the patterns, it is very important to realize that there are two sets of standards when interpreting blood chemistry.

One is the traditional range, which I call the sick range, which comes from the blood levels of everyone who went to the lab last year, including those people who have cancer or are dependent on oxygen, etc. These values are then averaged all together, and a bell shaped curve is created. The problem with this type of analysis is that it does not take into account what the optimal range for function is; it only determines if your body is in the disease state. Many people are having symptoms just outside these values but are considered normal by the medical profession. In order to make sense of why a person would have symptoms and still be considered "normal" is because the standard ranges are way too broad and they are using sick people to get their data. In order to achieve optimal function, we need data from healthy people. This second approach is called the functional range and is standardized throughout the country. The traditional range can change from state to state based on the level of ill health in that area of population.

For an example, let's look at TSH (thyroid stimulating hormone), which is made by the pituitary and tells the thyroid to make hormones.

Were all your tests normal?

Test	Optimal Ranges	Traditional "sick" lab ranges	Test Result & Interpretation
Glucose	85-100 mg/dl	65-125 mg/dl	82 - Hypoglycemia
TSH	1.4-3.0 ml U/L	0.3-5.7 ml U/L	4.2 - Hypothyroid
Cholesterol	150-200 mg/dl	<200 mg/dl	148 - Hormone imbalance
Triglycerides	75-100 mg/dl	<150 mg/dl	149 - Insulin resistance
Hemogloblin (Hgb)	F13.5-14.5 M14-15	12-16 gram /dl	13 - anemia

The functional range for TSH is 1.8 to 3.0, and the traditional range .3 to 5.7. In this case, this patient had classic low thyroid symptoms, which included fatigue, depression, cold hands, and cold feet, yet she was told "your lab tests are normal." We can see that based on the functional range she is clearly not normal and has subclinical thyroid problems.

It is very common for a patient to come into my office with a laundry list of health problems and yet they have been told by their doctor that everything is "normal." If you have heard this from your doctor, please don't accept that opinion until you have looked at your values using the functional range. Now that you understand this distinction we can move on and talk about the individual patterns.

Pattern #1: Primary Hypothyroid

Your thyroid has become lazy, likely due to some nutrient that your body is not getting. There are several nutrients that your body needs to make thyroid hormones: selenium, iodine, zinc, and vitamin A.

With this hypothyroid pattern your TSH would be above 3.0 and everything else would likely be in the functional range, with T4 and free T3 perhaps being low.

The functional range for total T4 is 6 to 12 and free T3 is 2.3 to 4.2

Pattern #2: Pituitary Suppression

The pituitary gland regulates thyroid hormone production in coordination with the hypothalamus. The pituitary gland is very sensitive to changes in body chemistry brought about by emotional stress and metabolic stress.

Emotional stress, blood sugar elevation, pain, chronic infection, poor diet, food allergies, or pregnancy can suppress the production of pituitary-produced TSH, causing a sluggish stimulus to the thyroid, the net result being low thyroid symptoms.

Blood test results would show a TSH level of less than 1.4, and the T4 may be less than 6.

Pattern #3: Underconversion

This pattern occurs due to adrenal-produced cortisol elevation.

High cortisol interferes with the conversion of T4 to T3. T3 is the thyroid hormone that has the biologic activity; if not enough is being converted you will have low thyroid symptoms. This pattern is often missed because doctors often **don't test** free floating T3 levels.

The gut and the liver are essential in converting T4 to T3. Functional problems with either of these organs can contribute to this pattern as well.

Blood chemistry in this pattern would show low free T3; the functional range is 2.3 to 4.2

We have talked a lot about the adrenal gland. Salivary testing is an easy, inexpensive, and accurate way to check the levels of cortisol and DHEA.

By looking at the graph below you will see that the production of cortisol changes from morning to night. The red lines show optimal ranges at different times of the day. The production of DHEA is relatively constant. Cortisol production is high in the morning and helps you wake up with energy to start your day. Cortisol production decreases as the day goes on and is lowest at bedtime. Cortisol and melatonin (the sleep hormone) oppose each other; it is important for cortisol to be low at night so melatonin can rise. Both low and high cortisol can contribute to fatigue.

Pattern #4: Overconversion

This pattern is the major high blood sugar pattern. When you are diabetic or have insulin resistance, this mechanism will cause your body to over convert T4 into T3. The excess hormone causes over time a resistance of the thyroid receptors and the net result, just like insulin, is the hormone does not get into the cell. As a result of too much hormone you end up with low thyroid symptoms. This pattern also results in over conversion of estrogen to testosterone via the liver. The high testosterone pattern in women is related to irritability, excessive facial hair and polycystic ovarian syndrome (P.C.O.S.). In a male overconversion an increase in estrogen production and loss of energy, libido and possibly the development of additional breast tissue.

The key to overcome this pattern is to correct the blood sugar problem.

Pattern #5: Increased Thyroid Binding

This pattern is associated with estrogen replacement therapy and oral contraception. When estrogen levels are too high, as is often the case when on replacement therapy like premarin and estrogen creams, this overstimulates the production of TBGs. Remember the thyroid binding globulins attach themselves to a lot of the free-floating thyroid hormones (and other hormones,) and once bound they don't let the free T3 go, so if we have many more of the these TBGs because of an increase in other hormones in the blood stream, we are going to have less unbound free T3, the net result low thyroid symptoms.

The key to address this pattern is to clear the body of excess estrogen. Taking birth control pills can cause this pattern.

The blood chemistry pattern you would look for is high levels of TBGs.

This marker is more often measured through an inverse marker called T3 uptake. If TBGs are high, T3 uptake is low. Functional range for T3 uptake is 28 to 34. Free T3 may be low as well, below 2.3.

Pattern #6: Thyroid

In this pattern all of the functional levels are in the ideal range and yet classic low thyroid symptoms persist. This can be a result of high homocysteine levels. Homocysteine is a toxic byproduct of protein metabolism that the body denatures to a harmless substance via B vitamins. Abnormal homocysteine levels can affect the production of myelin (fatty layer) around nerves and can affect neurotransmitter function.

The functional range is between 7 and 12.

There are several other physiological patterns that can disrupt thyroid dysfunction, but we have addressed the most common ones in this chapter.

If you want to know more about the non-autoimmune thyroid patterns, I would highly recommend a book entitled, *Why Do I Still Have Thyroid Problems When All My Lab Tests Are Normal?* By Dr. Datis Kharrazian.

Remember that you can have more than one pattern going on at the same time. The key is to do thorough testing and address all the mechanisms. The thyroid antibody testing findings trump everything else, and treatment becomes more complex. In the next chapter we will discuss how we address autoimmunity.

Take away: The key is to do thorough testing and address all the mechanisms. The thyroid antibody testing findings trump everything else, and treatment becomes more complex. In the next chapter we will discuss how we address autoimmunity.

Chapter 6. Addressing Autoimmunity

It must be a comprehensive approach.

To successfully address autoimmunity we have to determine if you have the condition. Tests can be ordered that can determine if you are making antibodies to thyroid enzymes (TPO), thyroid proteins (TG) and/or thyroid stimulating hormone receptors (TSI). Antibody tests for TPO or TG as well as TSI testing may help you determine if you have an autoimmune thyroid condition. It is also believed that your body may make antibodies to the thyroid receptor sites on the cells. Currently there is no test for this.

When you run the TPO, TBG, and TSI tests and the antibodies come back positive, you definitely have an autoimmune condition. However, if they come back negative it still does not rule out the condition.

Here's why. The TH2 system is responsible for antibody production, Hashimoto's is often a TH1 dominance, and in TH1 dominance the TH2 is suppressed so you may not be making many antibodies. So in this case you will have a false negative test.

Another issue that creates confusion is that the level of antibodies, whether it be just above range or very high, does not correlate with the severity of the symptoms. When the immune system attacks, it does so in waves; it attacks and relaxes. The fluctuation of antibodies on a daily basis makes it an unreliable marker to know if the condition is improving.

The biggest evidence that the patient is responding to care is that the symptoms are subsiding and other blood and saliva markers are improving.

Another important sign that you have developed Hashimoto's is that your TSH is up and down a lot and your thyroid medication dose keeps increasing. This pattern is evidence that you are losing more and more thyroid tissue from autoimmune attack. When the antibody test is not definitive, some doctors will use a three-day herbal challenge with substances that stimulate the TH1 system. Taking these products increases TH1 activity. If the patient were TH1 dominant, it would tend to aggravate the symptoms. If they were TH2 dominant, it would tend to make them feel better. If the patient is TH2 dominant, I can do the same herbal challenge with herbs that stimulate TH2 dominance.

When a patient that has persistent thyroid symptoms comes into my office, despite medication or other intervention, I assume they are autoimmune, because the research shows that nine out of ten times I will be right.

To successfully manage autoimmunity, we have to test for and address all the triggers, many of which we talked about in the last chapter.

#1. Find and defeat chronic infections.

Clues that you have chronic infections are shifts in your total white blood cell count. The functional range for the complete white blood cell count is 5.0 to 8.0. If you are lower or higher than that range, it is a sign your immune system is struggling. You may also have individual white cell markers that are out of the functional range.

Functional Range

Lymphocytes   25-40 percent of total WBC

If high, stressed immune system

If low, sluggish immune system

Neutrophils   40-60 percent

If high, immune compromise

If low, stressed immune system

Monocytes   less than 7 percent

If high, possible parasites, inflammation or infection

Eosinophils   less than 3 percent

If high, possible parasite or allergy

Basophils   0-1 percent

If high, possible parasite, inflammation

Once the infections are identified specific antimicrobial nutritional protocols will be followed to eliminate the infections from the body. Sometimes, although rarely, it is necessary to use prescription drugs to eliminate infections.

#2. Heal the gut.

Once we have eliminated chronic infections that are often found in the gut, we have to repair the damage to the intestinal lining. This means fixing the "leaks" in the gut. We do this with various substances such as **slippery elm, B vitamins, licorice root, bitter melon, glutamine, and pumpkin seed, among others.**

We often have to increase hydrochloric acid. HCL is produced by the stomach to digest protein and also protect you from getting an infection in the first place by keeping the acidity of the gut so high that foreign bugs can't live. Common symptoms of low HCL are bloating, feeling hungry one to two hours after meals, stomachaches and heartburn. Low HCL is one of the most common findings I see. HCL production declines with age and can be diminished due to lack of zinc, B vitamin, and irritation to the vagus nerve due to upper cervical spinal misalignments and cranial motion restriction.

It is interesting that many reflux/heartburn problems are greatly helped by increasing HCL, which seems odd since drugs (antacids) that stop HCL production also give relief. The problem is they don't address the underlying cause (as soon as you stop taking the drugs the symptoms come back). The acid blockers give temporary relief based on two mechanisms. First, they stimulate your stomach to push the undigested food out faster into the small intestine, which diminishes the time that the putrefying food stays in your stomach, and, second, the anti-acid pills not only arrest HCL production but they also diminish lactic acid that is produced from food that is not being broken down from a lack of HCL, so the symptoms improve temporarily. A lack of HCL will diminish overall digestive function impairing absorption of calcium and other important nutrients.

It may also be important to increase the levels of friendly bacteria, once the unfriendly bacteria is gone with probiotics.

#3. Eliminate inflammatory foods that create inflammatory immune responses.

Food allergies/sensitivities are a major factor in perpetuating autoimmune attack. The most common in order of predominance of reactive foods are gluten (a substance found in wheat, rye, and barley), dairy, eggs, soy, nightshades (potatoes, peppers, tomatoes, and eggplant), corn, rice, nuts, and legumes. You can have a sensitivity to any food, but these are the most common.

Why do you develop food allergies?

Sometimes it's genetic; your body does not produce the substance to metabolize dairy, gluten, or nightshades. Often, it is an acquired problem. You develop a chronic infection, and your intestinal membrane's healthy barrier breaks down, becoming porous, which lets undigested food and other foreign proteins leak into places where they don't belong. Your immune system responds to this invasion with escalating immune responses. This is the beginning of an acquired food sensitivity. Now every time you eat that food you have set up a new round of inflammation and autoimmune attack. HCL deficiencies, poor levels of friendly flora in the colon, as well as impaired gallbladder and liver function can contribute as well.

#4. Adrenal gland regulation.

An imbalance in your cortisol levels, both high levels and low levels, contributes to fatigue. If your DHEA levels are low, supplement DHEA to raise it. Low DHEA will decrease your ability to have adequate estrogen ad testosterone levels. High levels of cortisol are inflammatory and interfere with gland-to-gland communication and can also drive autoimmunity. Infection, food allergies, blood sugar problems, and emotional stressors are key drivers of adrenal problems.

#5 Regulate blood sugar.

Blood sugar and adrenal problems often occur together. Both low and high blood sugar result in not getting glucose into the cell for energy. Poor energy levels and brain fog can result. Elevated blood sugar, whether it be from diabetes or insulin resistance (prediabetes) stresses the brain and the nerves of the body.

Symptoms of low blood sugar: eating relieves fatigue (eating should only relieve hunger), don't feel like eating breakfast, feel lightheaded or irritable if missed meals, energy level drops in the midmorning and or midafternoon, strong cravings for sugar, irritability, and sluggish brain.

Solution: Eat small protein-based meals every two to three hours, decrease your sugar intake to prevent spikes and abrupt drops in blood sugar levels. Address all the above factors.

Symptoms of high blood sugar: Always want dessert or coffee after meals, feel tired after eating, waist girth is equal to or greater than your hip girth, difficulty losing weight, frequent urination.

Solution: Decrease sugar and carbohydrates consumption. Address all the above factors, start aerobic exercise. Paleo diet is excellent choice.

#6. Optimize vitamin D levels

Vitamin D is a critically important vitamin in the body and is especially central in regulating the immune system. Optimizing vitamin D levels helps your immune system to re-balance the TH1-TH2 shift. The minimum level for vitamin D is above 40. Some doctors advocate up to 80 or 90. It is quite common for vitamin D levels to be low; if that is the case we often give between 4,000 and 8,000 I.U. a day and then retest. If the vitamin D level is raised that is a good sign. If in spite of a high dose the level does not change, it can be a sign of liver dysfunction. Vitamin D is a hormone, not really a vitamin, and the liver is involved in recycling hormones in the body.

#7. Balance TH1 - TH2 shifts

Certain substances stimulate the TH1 and TH2 immune function.

TH1 stimulators are: astragalus, echinacea, licorice root, lemon balm, maitake mushrooms and pomegranate.

TH2 stimulators are: pine bark, grape seed extract, green tea, pycnogenol, caffeine, and reseveratrol.

Sometimes patients will try herbal supplements to help them feel better. If you felt worse doing so, you may have stimulated the wrong side of your immune system. If you have taken products from one of the two lists and felt better they may give you a clue as to which side your immune system has shifted.

The Liver

The liver performs many functions for the body. Detoxification of the body, especially the gut, is vital. The liver is involved in bile production and excretion, and along with the gall bladder is central in metabolizing fats. The liver is involved in activating enzymes, blood sugar storage, and converting T4 into useable T3.

It's an extremely busy organ. Any chronic health complaint could involve liver dysfunction. Correcting the digestive system is the highest priority, and then supporting the liver.

Anemia

Anemia is a deal breaker for any treatment program. When you have anemia, there are not enough healthy red blood cells to carry oxygen to the cells of the body; when your cells are starved for oxygen, basic cell function will be impaired. **In a later section where I will give you a list of tests you need to have done, it will also include testing for anemia.**

Graves' disease

What if you have Graves' disease? Graves' disease is hyperthyroidism.

Symptoms include: heart palpitations, anxiety, bulging eyeballs, inability to gain weight, insomnia, inward trembling, and increased resting pulse rate.

Graves' disease like Hashimoto's, is an autoimmune mechanism. The same autoimmune approach discussed earlier would be helpful.

Graves' disease would show a consistent low TSH of .5 or less. The TSH produced in the pituitary is being greatly suppressed because the body is being flooded with too much thyroid hormone.

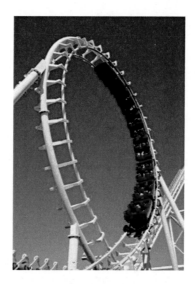

Now here is where it can get complicated.

Some Hashimoto's patients will have low and high thyroid symptoms at different times. Like a rollercoaster, the immune system mounts a massive attack, and a lot of thyroid hormone dumps into the blood stream, creating hyperthyroid symptoms so the immune response relaxes. Conversely, there can be low levels of thyroid hormones producing low thyroid symptoms; weight gain, fatigue, constipation, feeling cold, depression, and dry skin.

The determining factor to know the difference between Graves' (hyperthyroid) and Hashimoto's of the rollercoaster variety is that the symptoms are different:

TSH in Graves' (hyperthyroid stays low, less than .5)

In Hashimoto's TSH may be in range (1.8 to 3.0), for high above 3.0, or lower than 1.8 but not as low as .5 or TSH is unstable moving up and down.

Take away: *To be successful in healing your body and your thyroid, you have to address all the mechanisms whether you have autoimmunity or one of the six non-autoimmune patterns. Proper testing is the key. In a future chapter we will give you a list of all the tests that need to be done so that your condition can be managed successfully.*

Chapter 7. The Traditional Medical Approach to Thyroid Problems.

The current medical model for thyroid treatment in mainstream medicine is stuck in a time warp from the 1960s.

Today if you seek care from a traditional MD or endocrinologist, you will either get thyroid replacement, told you don't need replacement, or, if your condition can no longer be managed with thyroid replacement you will be urged to have your thyroid taken out if you have hypothyroidism. This very narrow approach does not take into account what the current research information is very clear about concerning thyroid problems. They are caused by multiple mechanisms, with the most common being autoimmunity. If this is true, why hasn't the medical profession updated their treatment models? Unfortunately this outdated approach is not likely to ever change. Why?

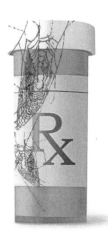

What does a medical doctor do? They perform surgery and write prescriptions. There is no prescription they can give you to address what is causing your thyroid autoimmunity and, no drug for leaky gut, food allergies or to restore proper adrenal dysfunction. These are the problems that functional/nutritional medicine is best at addressing. We also use different lab ranges. As a result, we find problems that the traditional range misses, that are considered normal but are not normal for optimal function. Medical doctors are trained to address diseases with medications but not to address the underlying symptoms that are causing these problems.

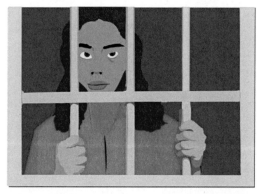

Outdated Medical Paradigm

Does this mean that you should stop taking thyroid replacement? Absolutely not! Before any suggestion for a change of prescription medication, a thorough evaluation must be done. Many patients who have had Hashimoto's for a long time but didn't know it may not have enough of their thyroid left to produce enough thyroid for the body and will need to continue with replacement. Those same patients will benefit greatly from care that is focused on the immune system which is the cause of the condition. **Thyroid replacement does not address autoimmunity.**

Natural Vs Synthetic Thyroid Hormone Replacement

This is a list of some of the common medications and the "natural" alternative thyroid substances.

Synthetic T4	Natural contains both T4 and T3 from pigs
Levothyroid	Armour
Levothroxine	Desiccated thyroid
Levoxyl	Naturethyroid
Synthyroid	Westroid (this product contains no fillers like glute or cornstarch

Synthetic T3

Cytomel

Synthetic T3 and T4

Thyroid

None of these substances address the autoimmunity that drives most thyroid problems.

However, they can be supportive if a lot of thyroid destruction has already occurred. The thyroid products that contain T3 will be helpful in those patients that have underconversion problems, as we discussed in chapter six.

Armour thyroid and other products that have T3 in them are very popular with natural medicine practitioners, however, in my experience since pig thyroid is closer to your own human thyroid there is a higher risk for the immune system to attack and make an autoimmune patient worse. Synthetic T4 does not seem to be as reactive as it is not as close to animal or human thyroid hormone.

Hashimoto's Patient Recovery

This patient came to my office with a lot of thyroid symptoms and was given thyroid hormones but always felt worse on them. She was frustrated and way too young to have life be so difficult. However, now with proper care she is off all medications and doing well. Watch this video to hear her story.

http://kirklandhealthinstitute.com/hashimotos-patient-recovery-video/

Chapter 8. How Do I Know If I Have Hashimoto's?

Health history and response to previous care are most important.

When patients come into my office with suspected thyroid symptoms or are already on thyroid hormones but still not feeling better, I assume that autoimmunity is the problem. Remember what the research shows. There are some cases that are not autoimmune and so we address any combination of the six factors that we discussed in chapter five.

A typical case presentation of Hashimoto's will appear with many of the following:

Health deteriorated after getting pregnant or after subsequent pregnancies. A lot of immune shifting occurs carrying the fetus.

Perimenopause brought on symptoms.

Puberty created onset.

Initially started thyroid replacement.

It did work at first, but now the dosage has to keep being increased to keep symptoms and TSH in range.

Your doctor has to lower and raise your replacement because your TSH is unstable.

Thyroid replacement made you feel worse, or it was helpful initially but now it's not working.

You tried natural thyroid (Armour); you felt worse.

You have tried herbal formulas, and you reacted badly to them.

Laboratory antibody testing revealed positive for any individual or combined TPO, TBG, or TSI.

If the antibodies are positive, you have confirmed autoimmunity. If they show negative, it does not rule out the condition.

Remember, the immune attack can wax and wane; doing the test during a symptomatic worsening may show a positive test. A challenge with provocative food sensitivities (gluten) or with herbal formulas may create a positive test that was previously negative. Herbal challenges with TH1 or TH2 herbs in which you feel much worse or better is a strong indication of autoimmunity. Oral challenges with these herbs should not create any reactions in a balanced immune system. The list of herbs is found in chapter six.

If you are TH1 dominant, your antibody-producing TH2 system may not be able to make sufficient antibodies to show a positive test.

Autoimmunity is going to be established by your medical history, family members who have similar problems, the onset of symptoms, your response to prior care that you have had, and/or your lab tests.

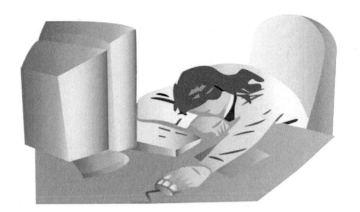

Chapter 9. The Brain-Thyroid Connection

There are many "cross talk" systems in the body.

Your nervous system and your glandular system talk to each other. Your individual glands all communicate to each other. Your immune system and your nervous system have a strong communication network. This is called "cross talk."

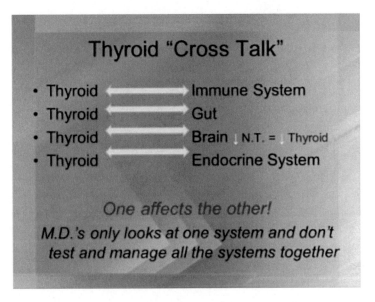

Every cell in your body needs thyroid hormone to function including your brain. Take this short brain test:

Is your memory noticeably becoming worse?

Are you having a hard time remembering names and phone numbers?

Is your ability to focus noticeably getting worse?

Has it become harder for you to learn things?

How often do you have a difficult time remembering appointments?

Is your temperament getting worse in general?

Are you losing your attention span endurance?

How often do you find yourself down or sad?

How often do you fatigue when driving compared to the past?

How often do you fatigue when reading compared to the past?

How often do you walk into rooms and forget why?

How often do you pick up your cell phone and forget why?

These are all signs of a brain that is going bad. They are signs of brain inflammation!

The autoimmune condition that you have is a condition where your body has intensifying inflammation. The brain, just like your other tissues, functions poorly when inflammation occurs. Inflammation weakens the neuron's ability to fire messages to the next neuron and so on until we have a global breakdown.

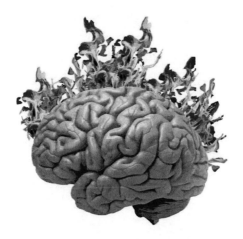

The autoimmune condition you may have is attacking other parts of your body as well. Research shows that in 50 percent of cases this is true.

> When you have an autoimmune condition, your gut is inflamed, and your immune cells, which are highly concentrated in your gut, are attacking like a loose cannon looking for anything that looks like the original offenders (infections, food sensitivities, heavy metals, etc.) in your body. These upset immune cells cross into the brain, bypassing the blood-brain barrier, and activate the immune cells in the brain called glial cells, which causes autoimmune damage to occur in the brain. Now you have just been taken down by a one-two punch; poor nervous system/brain function and metabolic disruption!

No wonder you feel terrible!

To get your brain functioning better, we have to do two things.

Address autoimmunity – see chapter six

Start brain rehabilitation therapy to restore function to the damaged areas. Yes, your brain can be rehabilitated just like a shoulder or knee. This phenomenon is known as "neuroplasticity." The brain is like a piece of silly putty that with specific stimulation therapies can be revitalized by strengthening damaged pathways and by making new connections.

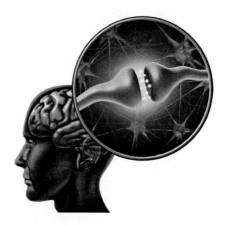

The healthcare specialty of functional neurology does just this. The amazing thing about it is that it happens so quickly. I have included some videos of patients after functional neurology care, pre and post visits. This therapy is also referred to as brain based therapy.

http://kirklandhealthinstitute.com/fibromyalgia-recovery-video/

http://kirklandhealthinstitute.com/brain-based-therapy-video/

Everyone knows how important the brain is, but it gets very little emphasis from traditional medicine. A medical neurologist is looking for dead nerves, tumors, etc., but is not trained to find and correct deficits that are causing symptoms that have not yet reached the state of disease.

Improving brain function is one of the most important things I do in my office.

Brain-thyroid success video:

http://kirklandhealthinstitute.com/brain-thyroid-success-video/

This patient came to my office with fatigue and brain problems so pervasive that she was fearful of losing her job. We confirmed she had Hashimoto's disease. Prior to our care she was on synthyroid medication, which over time stopped helping, and she also did poorly on her neurological exam. Watch her video to see how much better she is doing today.

Chapter 10. The Brain-Thyroid-Pain Connection

A healthy brain helps dampen the brain response.

I see a lot of chronic-pain patients in my office. One of the things that we screen all these patients for is a thyroid problem. If you have low thyroid function one of the symptoms you can have is body aches and pain. If the pain is throughout the whole body and you have difficulty with sleep, this is called fibromyalgia. Fibromyalgia is thought to be a problem in which the brain loses the ability to dampen pain. A healthy brain should be able to dampen pain. The fibromyalgia patients that I see often have this brain imbalance in the part of the brain called the sympathetic nervous system, or the "fight or flight" system. This system is permanently switched on. In order to help these patients, we have to balance the brain with functional neurology. These patients often have secondary mechanisms to promote inflammation on the metabolic side as well, including thyroid, adrenal, blood sugar, food allergies, and autoimmunity.

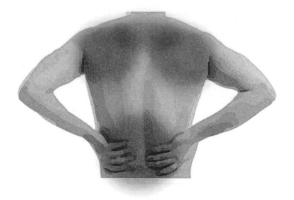

Fibromyalgia-Thyroid Testimonial

This patient came to my office with fibromyalgia symptoms. She was very tired, so much so that she had to have three alarm clocks set in her bedroom at slightly different times to insure that she would eventually get out of bed in the morning!

See how she is doing today:

http://kirklandhealthinstitute.com/resolved-thyroid-symptoms-video/

Chapter 11. Weight Loss and the Thyroid

Inability to lose weight even on a low-calorie diet is a red flag for thyroid evaluation.

If you have a weight problem and you have had challenges getting it under control, there are many variables that could be at the root of the problem. The two most common are high blood sugar and thyroid dysfunction.

When your blood sugar rises, the receptor sites that respond to insulin become resistant. The net effect is you can't get glucose into the cell, so the body coverts that energy into fat and stores it for future use. The excess fat gets stored around your midsection, and your abdomen will eventually become wider than your hips.

You will also often want to have sweets after a meal because the sugar is not getting into the cell, so the net result is you want more sugar. It's a vicious cycle that creates more resistance, more craving, and more weight gain. The conversion of glucose to fat takes a lot of energy, so you may also feel tired after you eat.

The solution for rising blood sugar is to change your food selections. Switch the percentage of foods to favor more protein and fewer carbohydrates. Stop eating the foods that spike blood sugar. These are grains and anything with added sugar. Eat low-glycemic vegetables and fruits, like asparagus, fennel, cucumber, beets, greens, lettuce (any kind), chard, bok choy, onion, tomatoes, cabbage, radishes, celery, spinach, apples, oranges, grapefruits, strawberries, and lemons.

Lowering your blood sugar will help recondition your cell receptors so you can burn glucose and reengage your body's ability to mobilize your fat stores so you can lose weight that you have been storing in your fat cells for so long. Lowering your blood sugar will also keep you from overconverting your T4 into too much free T3, overwhelming your receptors with too much hormone and creating a resistance to thyroid hormones. The net effect is low thyroid symptoms. See chapter five.

Low thyroid function causes weight gain and can create an inability to lose weight even on a low-calorie diet. When the thyroid is the cause, your metabolic thermostat is turned down so low that you aren't burning calories. This is why many thyroid sufferers also feel cold. The pilot light is so low it is not able to light the whole furnace.

I have had many patients who have not been able to lose weight because of a thyroid problem that was not found or managed properly.

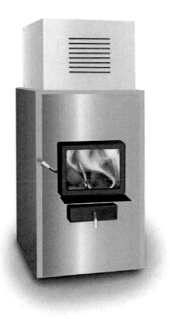

Case study: this female patient came to me because of an inability to lose any weight despite vigorous workouts with a personal trainer for over one year! She had afternoon fatigue as well. Not only is her energy level much better but she also has finally lost a lot of weight as well!

Watch her story!

http://kirklandhealthinstitute.com/thyroid-weightloss-video/

Chapter 12. Goiters and Goitrogenic Foods

An often misunderstood concept

It is often believed that if you have a goiter, (thickening of the thyroid gland tissue), it is caused by an iodine deficiency, and that if you eat certain foods this can also cause a goiter.

An enlarged thyroid gland can be caused by two main issues:

1) Swelling due to diffuse inflammation or "thyroiditis", this swelling can be from:

A) Auto-immune attack, Hashimoto's. This swelling would increase and decrease based on the waxing and waning effect of the immune system attacking the thyroid. This swelling would be painless to the touch.

B) Local thyroid infection which would be accompanied by fever and would be painful to the touch. In both of these cases the whole gland is swollen.

2) Swelling due to a goiter, a thickening of the tissue around the thyroid gland, which does not change in size. The thyroid tissue enlarges because the TSH level is too high which overstimulates thyroid tissue growth, (HCG can also cause this). TSH elevation is often due to Hashimoto's and can also be from an iodine deficiency, but this is a very rare situation in our country due to iodized salt and readily available fresh vegetables.

You can also have a solitary swelling in one area of the thyroid unlike the diffuse swelling discussed above. Solitary swelling can be from a benign cyst, nodules or from malignancy. The key factor is to differentiate via thyroid ultrasound to determine the cause of the solitary swelling, and see if your whole thyroid has thickened (goiter).

Goitergenic Substances

Certain foods, drugs and chemicals can interrupt iodine uptake in the thyroid gland. Foods such as strawberries, peaches, spinach, Brussel sprouts, cauliflower, kale and cabbage in very large amounts can disrupt iodine absorption. This should not be a concern unless you are juicing these foods in large quantities.

Medications that may promote goiter:

Anti-thyroid medications (methimasole, Tapazol, propylthiouracil): used for hyperthyroid patients

Sulfonamides: used to prevent the growth of bacteria in the body

Amiodarone (cardarone): used as an anti-arrhythmic agent

Ethionamide (Trecator): used as an antibiotic for the treatment of tuberculosis

Aminosalicylate Sodium (Tubasal): used an anti-infective for the treatment of tuberculosis

Lithium: used for bipolar disorders, depression, anxiety, cluster headaches and migraines

Aminoglutethimide: used for the treatment of Cushing's syndrome and other endocrine disorders that produce excess hormones (glucocorticoids, mineral corticoids, estrogen, androgens)

Salofalk: used for the treatment of ulcerative colitis

Environmental compounds that may promote goiter

Mercury, Arsenic and potentially other heavy metals

Nitrates

Pesticide compounds

Points to consider when you have an enlarged thyroid gland

I encourage thyroid patients with enlarged thyroid glands to consider the following points:

1. If you have been diagnosed with a goiter, make sure you ask for an ultrasound. Many doctors misdiagnose painless autoimmune thyroiditis as a goiter. A thyroid ultrasound delivers a clear and proper diagnosis.

2. If you have an actual goiter, please test your TSH to see whether the goitrogenic mechanism is still active. If TSH is elevated please test TPO and TGB thyroid antibodies to rule out Hashimoto's, the most common cause of goiter. If your TSH is normal, then something in the past caused your goiter.

3. Be cautious of health care providers who immediately assume iodine deficiency when you have a goiter. They will place you on iodine and be shocked to see your goiter size not change. Remember, goiter tissue is permanent tissue enlargement. It can only be reduced with excess thyroid hormones to induce atrophy or surgery, not iodine.

4. If you have painless autoimmune thyroiditis, pay careful attention to any mechanisms that cause it to swell, which can indicate exacerbation of autoimmunity. The most common triggers are food intolerances, stress, overtraining, overworking, and lack of sleep. You can use topical glutathione cream directly into your thyroid gland and see if it reduces your swelling. [4] Footnote taken from Dr. K's News Nov 12 2013

Chapter 13. More about Iodine?

Savior or villain?

It is not uncommon to read information in books and on the Internet touting the benefits of iodine. It is true that your thyroid gland needs adequate amounts of iodine to make T4 and T3 thyroid hormones. Iodine was added to table salt many years ago to help prevent iodine deficiency. Despite consuming iodized salt, it still might be possible that you could be deficient. If you suspect you are low in iodine, you can have a urine iodine challenge test. As a note of caution, it may not be wise to supplement with iodine without testing or professional supervision due to the fact that research has shown that iodine can fuel autoimmunity. Here's why. Supplementing with iodine stimulates the production of TPO. If you have Hashimoto's, TPO is often the site of autoimmune attack so every time TPO production is stimulated, the immune system, which perceives TPO as a foreign invader to be eradicated, goes into attack mode. This would cause your TPO antibody level to rise, making you feel worse.

Chapter 14. Heavy Metal Toxicity and Methylation Problems

Two important problems with any chronic condition

Heavy metal toxicity

We are all exposed to toxins, it is part of living in this modern world. Your body has mechanisms to eliminate toxins such as heavy metals, chemicals and exogenous hormones or xenoestrogens through the liver, bowels, kidneys, lungs and skin. If our exposure is greater, or our detox mechanisms are sluggish, our toxicity load increases. The term "heavy metals" describes metals that are higher on the periodic elemental chart than essential metals like zinc, copper, selenium, magnesium, and manganese.

Oftentimes, the vague symptoms produced by heavy metal toxicity are mistakenly misdiagnosed as incurable chronic conditions (ie. autoimmune disorders, neurological disorders, peripheral neuropathy, chronic pain syndromes, etc.). Heavy metal toxicity has a direct effect on healing, tissue repair, growth, genes-RNA and DNA, hormones, brain and nerves, liver, lungs, GI, reproductive organs, heart, thyroid, kidneys, adrenals, pancreas and body metabolism. Basically, heavy metal toxicity affects every bodily function. The most common heavy metals that humans are exposed to are aluminum, arsenic, cadmium, lead, and mercury.

Heavy metals are found in everyday existence and are frequently hard to avoid entirely. Most people can excrete toxic heavy metals from the body successfully. However, some people—especially those who suffer from chronic conditions—cannot excrete them efficiently enough, and a build-up occurs. Recent research also reveals that those who cannot excrete heavy metals efficiently appear to be genetically predisposed to this condition. Research has also shown that the APO-E 4/3 and 4/4 genotypes are the worst excretors of heavy metals. Those with this version of APO-E protein—abundant in the cerebral spinal fluid surrounding the brain—will have the highest affinity for becoming ill from exposure to neuro-toxic heavy metals, especially mercury when it is present in combination with others. [6]

It is important to have your heavy metal levels analyzed. Unfortunately, in our toxic world, high levels of heavy metals are common. What are the consequences of having high levels of mercury, lead or another heavy metal? As I mentioned before, heavy metal toxicity can lead to a host of neurological problems including dementia, brain fog, Alzheimer's, and Parkinson's disease.

The human body does not like heavy metals 'floating' around in the serum. Therefore, it tightly binds them up primarily in fat tissue. However, if a person with high heavy metal levels loses a significant amount of weight, especially in the fatty areas of the body, they can release a toxic load of heavy metals into the serum. Unfortunately, neurological tissue can also bind heavy metals. If the fat tissues are saturated or there is not enough fat to bind heavy metals, neurologic tissue will store the metals. Studies have shown that small amounts of mercury can destroy nerve fibers.

What can you do? The first step is to work with a health care practitioner who is knowledgeable about heavy metals. The doctor should know how to test for and how to treat heavy metal toxicity. I can guarantee you that nearly all physicians neither have the knowledge nor the training to do this. I suggest finding a holistic health care practitioner who does have the appropriate education to identify and treat heavy metal toxicity. [7]

I routinely test my patients for heavy metal toxicities using urine testing. A simple blood test will not suffice, as I mentioned previously, the body does not like heavy metals 'floating' around in the blood stream. There are many different products that patients can take orally to bind to the heavy metals and then excrete. The product I use the most is called "Chloroenergy". Chloroenergy is a green algae product that detoxes heavy metals and is tolerated by most people.

Below are some symptoms that may be associates with specific heavy metals and sources of exposure. [8]

ALUMINUM

Any amount aluminum is too much!!

Aluminum toxicity is associated with Alzheimer's and Parkinson's disease, behavioral/learning disorders such as ADD, ADHD, and autism.

High levels of aluminum have been found in the hair of delinquent, psychotic, and pre-psychotic boys, and in juvenile offenders.

Aluminum has neurotoxic effects at high levels, but low levels of accumulation may not elicit immediate symptoms.

Early symptoms of aluminum burden may include fatigue, headache, and other symptoms.

Aluminum is a heavy metal that displaces your other good minerals, such as magnesium, calcium, zinc, and phosphorus.

Research has proven that fluoride and fluoridation (in tap water) increases the absorption of aluminum.

Symptoms

Alzheimer's

Parkinson's

Behavioral/learning disorders such as ADD, ADHD and autism

Fatigue

Headache

Sources

Anti-perspirants

Emulsifiers in processed cheese

Table salt – anti-caking compound

Aluminum cookware

Bleaching agent in white flour

Buffered aspirin

Some toothpaste

Dental fillings

Cigarette filters

Contaminated water

Aluminum cookware

Antacids

Vaccines

Some baking sodas

Baking powder

Some breath mints

Some skin lotions

Some cosmetics

Aluminum foil

Canned goods

ARSENIC

Ingestion of large amounts of soluble Arsenic compounds effect the myocardium, causing death within a few hours.

The current EPA standard for arsenic in public water systems is 10 ppb, reduced from 50ppb in 2006. The standard applies only to drinking water sources that serve more than 20 people.

Arsenic, Water, Cancer

Even small amounts of arsenic might cause cells to lose some of their ability to repair genetic damage!

The results help explain why arsenic contamination in drinking water can lead to certain cancers.

Without the ability to repair its DNA, a cell could be vulnerable to damage from pollutants such as cigarette smoke.

Dartmouth Medical School, International Journal of Cancer 4/2003 Symptoms

Symptoms

Bone marrow depression

Skin discolorations

Liver and kidney degeneration

Agitation

Confusion

Vomiting

Eczema

Hair loss

Respiratory issues

Anemia

Neurological symptoms

Cancers

Learning impairment

Malaise

Diarrhea

Muscle weakness

Stomach pain

Sources

Tobacco smoke

Metal smelting

Production of glass	Ceramics
Artificial colors	Insecticides
Fungicides	Herbicides
Drinking water	Wood treatments

Cadmium

Cadmium (Cd) is a toxic, heavy metal with no positive metabolic function in the body and is relatively rare but more toxic than lead.

Moderately high cadmium levels are consistent with hypertension, while very severe cadmium toxicity can cause hypotension.

Cadmium absorption is reduced by zinc, calcium and selenium.

Alkaline Phosphatase is commonly elevated with Cadmium toxicity.

Cadmium toxicity is common among welders and construction workers (cement dust).

Contamination may come from perms, dyes, bleach, some hair sprays, and can cause false highs for Cd.

Symptoms

Hypertension	Fatigue
Muscle and joint pain	Low back pain
Atherosclerosis	Affects the
kidneys	
Lungs	Testes
Arterial walls	Bones

Interferes with many enzymatic systems   Leads to anemia

Protein and glucose in urine   Depletes calcium, phosphorus, and zinc

Sources

Refined foods (white flour, white sugar, etc.)   Acidic drinks

Super phosphate fertilizers   Some cola drinks

Tap water   Atmospheric pollution in the burning of coal and petroleum products

Margarine   Canned foods

Cigarette smoke and dyes   FD&C colors

Perms   Dyes

Bleach and some hair sprays

Cement dust (common among welders and construction workers)

Lead

Physiologically, the renal, nervous, reproductive, endocrine, immune and hemopoietin systems are affected.

Sub-toxic oral exposure to lead and cadmium increases the susceptibility to bacterial and viral infections.

Lead is known to damage the kidney, the liver and the reproductive system, as well as to interfere with bone marrow function, basic cellular processes and brain functions.

It is known to be responsible for convulsions, abdominal pain, paralysis, temporary blindness, extreme pallor, loss of weight and appetite, constipation, and numerous other problems.

Lead causes nerve and mental problems, especially affecting learning ability in children.

It was reported that the IQs of middle-class children dropped five to seven points after lead exposure, and Moon, et. al., demonstrated that lead levels also related to decreased visual and motor performance.

Lead interferes with utilization of calcium, magnesium, vitamin D, and zinc.

Symptoms

Abdominal pain	Colic
Severe and repeated vomiting	Irritability
Hyperactivity	Anorexia
Loss of appetite	Mental disturbances
Anemia	Gastric distress
Fatigue	Weight loss
Headaches	Vertigo
Tremor	Joint pain
Poor coordination	Neuritis
Poor memory	Constipation

Interferes with calcium, magnesium, vitamin D, and zinc

Source

Lead based paints	Crystal

Ceramics

Food crops

Water contamination

Some fertilizers

Canned food

Artificial colors

Industrial pollution

Methylation

Methylation is the process that involves the biologically activation of B12 and B9 and the donating of carbon molecules (CH3) to the methylation pathway. The methylation pathway is a very important cellular mechanism involved in detoxification, inflammation and neurotransmitter function, it stimulates good gene function and suppresses bad gene function. This process of methylation happens billions of times in every cell and the byproducts of which the body needs for other functions. If the methylation process is not working properly it will result in liver, digestive, immune, mood, neurological, and blood sugar problems. The big picture is that it can affect just about everything, the list of diseases and syndromes is very long so it's very important to make sure this mechanism is working properly. Genetic mutations can occur causing problems with this important process. The good news is that despite genetic disruption, targeted nutritional support can help ease the burden of methylation dysfunction.

Blood testing can determine if we have genetic defects that are affecting the methylation pathway. Single Nucleotides Polymorphisms or SNiP's can be tested for, because they relate to the MTHRF enzyme. This enzyme is key in taking dietary vitamin B-12 and B-9 and converting those vitamins to useable forms (Methylfolate, Methylcobalamin) that the methylation pathway needs to function properly. MTHRF defects are important to test for; you can have either the C677T and or the

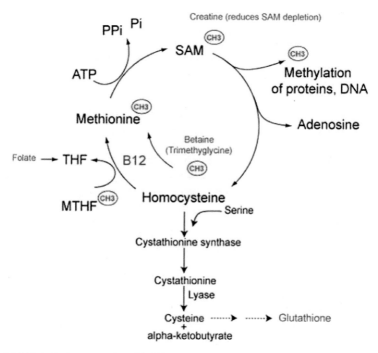

A1298C defect. Both will affect your conversion to the bioavailable form of Vitamin B9 and B12, and will impair your methylation cycle.

You can compensate for this defect my supplementing with the pre-methylated form of the vitamins bypassing the defect and helping your methylation cycle perform more normally. There are other genetic tests that can be performed for other metabolic problems but that discussion is beyond the scope of this book. You can have all your SNiP's tested at https://www.23andme.com/

Chapter 15. My Secret Weapon

The tool that the best doctors I know use.

Applied kinesiology (A.K.) is a holistic approach to health that uses the feedback response from the body via manual muscle testing. Applied kinesiology was started by Dr. George Goodheart of Detroit, Michigan, in the 1960s. Dr. Goodheart was uniquely famous for helping people who had stumped other doctors. He was the first chiropractor that treated Olympic athletes at Lake Placid in 1980.

Others doctors have taken Dr. Goodheart's discoveries and utilized the muscle-testing response to address many areas of health, emotional problems, nutritional imbalances, learning problems, and structural and muscular problems. When you are using manual muscle testing you are accessing the nervous system. To resist against a force applied to the muscle, the brain spinal cord and the peripheral nerves are all engaged. The acupuncture system and, the nutritional and the emotional status are all monitored by the nervous system. When a muscle tests weak, it may be due to any of these factors. Correcting these factors will reengage the nervous system, and the muscle will test noticeably stronger. Muscle testing can be used to challenge the body with various substances to see how the muscle (nervous system) is affected.

For more information on AK watch this video:

http://kirklandhealthinstitute.com/applied-kinesiology-video/

There are many issues that relate to chronic health conditions in which all of our labs give us good information, but there are still often unanswered questions.

Unfortunately, blood tests cannot often tell us what specific infections a patient has and cannot tell us what antimicrobial nutritional support will help the body get rid of the infections.

AK is very helpful in this situation.

What food allergies does the patient have? Nightshades are a common one. Apha-solaine is a substance found in all nightshades, including tomatoes, potatoes, peppers, eggplant, and goji berries. The alpha-solaine in nightshades can cause joint pain, skin rashes, and other symptoms. There is no blood test for this. What if there is an emotional component to a physical symptom? This is a very common occurrence. AK can help determine that and address other issues as well. AK can give doctors important information about the body, leading to a corrective action.

Combining muscle testing, neurological examination, and laboratory analysis has helped me solve the tough cases that come to my office. It is not unusual for a patient to have been to four or five doctors, sometimes more, before they find my office.

Chapter 16. What Is the Next Step for You?

This makes all the difference.

Finding the right doctor is the most important piece of your recovery. The doctor you trust with your recovery must be trained in functional medicine and have a thorough understanding of the autoimmune component to thyroid problems. They should have a successful track record of helping Hashimoto's/thyroid patients with either written or video testimonials.

Your doctor should also be trained in functional neurology so if your brain needs rehabilitation they know what to do.

Better yet, are they an expert in using applied kinesiology to augment the information they have from the labs and neurological findings?

Once you find this doctor, these tests should be ordered:

Comprehensive metabolic profile

Hepatic panel, including cholesterol and triglycerides

Complete WBC count with differential

Iron and ferritin levels

Vitamin D level

LDH

Homocysteine level

Phosphorus

Uric acid

Full thyroid panel, including, TSH, T4, free T3, T3 uptake, thyroid AB's TPO, TBG, TSI is optional

Adrenal saliva stress Index, including four cortisol readings, DHEA levels, and, if necessary, you can add female or male hormone panel. For females, this would check for the three estrogens, testosterone, and progesterone. I use Diagnos-Techs Labs.

http://www.diagnostechs.com/

Food allergy testing: If using a lab, I believe Cyrex Laboratories has the most accurate testing because they are testing for multiple immune markers like IGG and IGA, while most labs only test one marker.

https://www.cyrexlabs.com/

Key points from this book

You still suffer because thorough testing has not been done to discover the causes of your poor health.

You likely have an autoimmune condition that your doctor has not tested for and does not know how to address.

If you are autoimmune, your condition is progressive.

Combining neurological and metabolic therapy gives you the best chance for maximum improvement.

With proper care, the symptoms of autoimmunity and low thyroid function can be reversed.

You need to find a doctor who is an expert in this area to help you recover.

Chapter 17. It's Time to Get Your Health Back!

It's the opportunity of a lifetime!

Take some time and seriously consider these important questions:

How has your condition affected your job, family relationships, finances, or other activities? What have you given up on doing again?

What has your condition already cost you in money, sleep, and happiness?

If your condition does not improve, what do you anticipate your life to be like in one to three years?

What worth do you place on getting your health back if I can help you?

What we need from you:

For our office to be able to accept you as a patient, you have to be able to commit to three things.

You will have to be willing to make serious lifestyle changes, changing poor habits, including what you eat. If we find gluten sensitivity, which is very common, you will have to be 100 percent off gluten. We will teach you how to do this and what you can safely eat.

You must take complete accountability for your health. To get from where you are to where you want to be, you're going to have to take charge of your health.

The insurance model will pay for care that keeps you dependent on medications for the rest of your life! Unfortunately, it won't pay for the care that will investigate why you are sick and give you the care you need to get your life back. It's not fair, but that is the way it is. If you want life-changing care, you are going to have to pay for it out of your own pocket. Insurance and Medicare will only cover a small portion of your care.

We have made our care affordable so that 90 percent of patients can get the care they need.

People spend money every day on things insurance does not pay for: cars, vacations, jewelry, and electronics. These businesses are prospering despite no insurance reimbursement. Why? Because people want those things!

Your health and happiness is worth much more than anything. Taking care of your mind and body is the best investment you will ever make.

Committed patients can regain their health and make their dreams come true. Watch this video of a patient who was only able to work four hours a day due to her health problems. She bought a one-hundred-year-old house that she was losing hope of ever being able to renovate, turning it into her dream bed and breakfast. See how she is doing today after only a month of care!

http://kirklandhealthinstitute.com/brain-thyroid-auto-immune-recovery-video/

What if you live out of the area? No problem. You can go to www.lifechangingcare.com and find a qualified doctor to help you.

If you still are some distance from a qualified doctor, I also do distance consulting for patients via Skype and e-mail.

There is no reason not to get better!

References

[1] Christopher Murray, M.D, PhD, director of WHO's Global Programme on Evidence for Health Policy.

[2] Bailliere's Clin. Endocrinal Metabolism 1988 Aug; 2 (3): 591-617

[3] Acta Biomed 2003 Apr: 74 (1): 9-33 Ibid 52 percent have polyendocrine problems

Datis Kaharrazian DHSc, DC, MS. *Why Do I Still Have Thyroid Symptoms When All My Lab Tests Are Normal?* Morgan James 2010 ISBN 978-1-60037-670-2

[4] Dr. K's News Nov 12 2013

[5] *You Can Beat Thyroid Problems* by Dr. Michael Johnson

[6] *Why You Need to Identify and Treat Heavy Metal Toxicity,* Dr. Brownstein's July 10th 2015 blog

[7] *You Can Beat Thyroid Problems* by Dr. Michael Johnson

[8] *You Can Beat Thyroid Problems* by Dr. Michael Johnson

Do you want to learn more about Dr. Taggart's practice and healing techniques? Please go to http://kirklandhealthinstitute.com/

E-mail: DrT@KirklandHealthInstitute.com

Feel free to ask any questions; there is no charge.

If you are interested in visiting Dr. Taggart's office for an initial consultation, please call 425-821-1101. If you live in an area beyond Seattle, WA, USA, a phone or Skype consultation can be scheduled.

?

Made in the USA
San Bernardino, CA
18 January 2016